Walking in my st

Finding bala

Mummy

It's your turn to shine. Please bring forth all that is in you ma.

Aramide

Copyright © 2019 Aramide Fadiora.

All rights reserved.

Cover design by JOScreative

Book design by Swiss Graphics

No part of this book can be reproduced in any form or by written, electronic or mechanical, including photocopying, recording, or by any information retrieval system without written permission in writing by the author.

Published by Independent Publishing Network

Edited by Aquile Publishing

Printed in Great Britain

Although every precaution has been taken to prepare this book, the publisher and author assume no responsibility for errors or omissions. Neither is any liability assumed for damages resulting from information contained herein.

ISBN 978-178972-810-1

ACKNOWLEDGEMENT

I want to thank God for His grace, mercy and steadfast love from the first breath. I owe Him every ounce of my life and all.

A special thank you to my beautiful family and all the fantastic people (friends and church members) around me who have been so supportive and caring in ways I could never have imagined. Thank you Sabina Ben Salmi and Roxanne St Clair for allowing me to stand on your shoulders, you made this possible, and I am ever so grateful. I want to thank spiritual fathers and mothers for your profound insights. A special thank you to Ma, a woman of high strength and wisdom and over 45 years of marriage. Thank you for sharing your insight into marriage and for prayerfully supporting me. A special thank you to Chief (Pastor Kolade Adebayo-Oke) for writing the foreword. Your humility and impact on our generation are phenomenal. I am grateful for the life of Pastor Joe Wole who believed in me and launched me into ministry and patiently mentored me over the years. A million thank you's to AdeY for everything that I cannot share in this book. You are truly amazing, and I am grateful that you are part of my journey. I cannot but mention my spiritual home and family, GH London. I am truly blessed to be part of this wonderful church.

Finally, my beautiful kids for making life colourful.

FOREWORD

I have found the book 'Walking in my stilettos' very interesting, refreshing and delightful to read. The writer, using very simple and direct expressions, delivers a very deep message in practical ways. I have been privileged to have known her for many years as a person with a genuine heart for God and others, and also as a straight talker. She doesn't disappoint here. The core message of this book is for the reader to find and identify their purpose in life and to walk in it. She has beautifully woven the message with reference to her and others' experiences in life, and also with reference to wise sayings from the Holy Bible.

This book is relevant to people of all age groups and circumstances. There is so much wisdom to gain from a read of it. The way the message is presented in such an inspiring and matter of fact, yet compassionate, fashion, would inspire the reader to read it again and again. The Holy Bible, in Proverbs 4:7, says "Wisdom is the principal thing; therefore get wisdom: and with all your getting, get understanding". This book ticks the right boxes in this respect.

The book 'Walking in my stilettos' in many useful ways encourages the reader to develop the qualities of character, a love for God and others, and a willingness to trust and obey God. When these qualities are being developed inside us by the Holy Spirit, God can use us in big or small ways to accomplish His will on earth and impact others positively. Indeed, we are informed that, despite adversities and challenges in life, it is still very possible for us to discover our God-given purpose and successfully walk in our stilettos. And that will help us to find the right balance in our everyday life.

Pastor Kolade Adebayo-Oke

Dedicated to

Mummy and every wonder woman

CHAPTER 1

HAPPY FEET

A few years ago, while I was reading the classic story of Cinderella with my daughter, she sat and listened carefully. I noticed the questioning look on her face and asked her what she was thinking about. She then asked why Cinderella was the only size four in town. She reminded me I had called someone's feet very small at size four. I wasn't even aware she was listening to everything I was saying. Nothing in the Cinderella story suggested Cinderella was a size four. More importantly, her question, as naïve as it was, had me puzzled for some time too, and that question will form the basis of this book. It is this notion I set to look at, not from the wisdom of a four-year-old, but to draw on both physical and spiritual perspectives to provoke you to search for your lost shoe.

Midwives used to encourage that we reuse old clothes and pass me downs as a way of saving money. This is very true considering children can outgrow clothes quicker than you would like to imagine. They did, however, stress that shoes should not be passed down for hygiene reasons and, more importantly, to allow the new baby's feet to grow naturally. When I thought about this, it made perfect sense as it takes time for the feet to break into new shoes. The shoe ultimately responds to the uniqueness of the owner in the shape, length and walking habits. This process of "breaking in" does not last forever, but sometimes the process can be painful. The pain can be bad enough to give you nasty corns on the feet or make the feet slightly swollen. However, the more you use it, the quicker the feet and shoes adapt to each other.

Although rarely considered one of the most essential body parts, the many connections of muscles, ligaments and tendons provide balance and motion in the feet. It gives the relationship between our body and surface through gravity. Your ability to stand, move, run and exercise are all functions of the feet that your body depends on every day. The foot is one organ that if it's working fine, you don't think about it until it fails or hurts. A young man was discussing how frightened he was of going to the dentist, and had not been for over 15 years and swore he'd never go. His wisdom tooth played up a few months later, and he called to ask for a right dentist that would be gentle and willing to see him the same day. Money was no longer an issue because the pain was excruciating. Sometimes, it's so easy to take so much for granted because it's there and we expect it to work. What do you do when you have something available but not useful, present but useless? That can be very frustrating. That is the experience of the man that was born lame from his mother's womb in John 5. Imagine being immobile for 38 years!

The feet amongst their two primary duties bear the brunt of our weight and protect against the impact of different surfaces. The feet are so crucial because of the connection they have with all the other organs. I find it incredible that someone can experience healing and relaxation in corresponding parts of the body by applying pressure to areas of the feet through reflexology. Our feet, therefore, protect other organs in the body.

Growing up, I preferred loafers and flats rather than stilettos until I was encouraged by a friend to wear high heels. Naturally, I objected because I am blessed vertically and horizontally and did not want to be taller than everyone else by wearing heels. After a while, I succumbed and bought a pair. It was painful! Now, some women are so blessed they can wear the highest heels and walk on the cloud with them, but I struggled significantly in heels initially. My walking became noticeably slower, my body more tensed for fear of falling from an unnecessary height.

And my focus shifted to my feet rather than walking head high. My toes were often so squashed I'd have to apply cold press to numb the pain. The questions I'd often ask myself were "who asked me" or "is it by force" as I reeled into self-pity. On a personal note, I cannot take walking for granted. I had a period of not being able to walk when I was younger, and walking is one thing I am most grateful for. The full use of any body part is a privilege, not a right. But the shoe I buy is a choice, a means of adding value and beautifying myself to look and feel a certain way.

Thinking about this, it seems so ironic that many have so mastered someone's shoes and walking habits that they become strangers to the one life intended for them.

Looking back at my daughter's question, I realized that what the fairy godmother gave Cinderella was unique to her. It wasn't the size that mattered but the fit of the shoe. You can line up a hundred people of the same size, and give them the same brand of footwear. The fit will vary from one person to another, and the way the shoe adapts to each person will also be different.

Many people go through life, trying to break into shoes already broken into by someone else. They subject themselves to pain and dilemma that life did not intend for them. What is more alarming is that we inevitably pass that same shoe down to our children, or from one sibling to the other.

As we go through this book, I hope that the pages uncover and address areas where the shoe is pinching or hurting. The ultimate goal is to get your feet back into alignment and let yourself do what you were naturally designed to do.

CHAPTER 2

THE SOUL
Go back to the beginning

The Greek word for soul is psuche or psychi, while in Hebrew nephesh.

What I find fascinating is that the word psychology is derived from psychi and psychology studies the human mind, its processes and functions.

Human beings comprise three distinctive parts; the spirit, the soul and the body. The spirit, translated as pneuma (in Greek), is the unseen that is ever searching for meaning and purpose and ultimately in search of the divine and spiritual. It is a force or wind. If you have ever been privileged to see someone pass away, sometimes you might notice a change of breathing at the final moment. For some, it can be quite rigorous as they struggle to hold on to that last breath, while for some, it is just a deep breath. That very breath is the spirit, the difference between whether someone is alive or dead. The most noticeable thing is the change in colour immediately someone passes away and the sudden coldness in the hands. The spirit cannot be overlooked because it feeds and sustains the soul. Even as I write this, I am reminded that the very breath I sometimes take for granted, someone else is struggling to hold on to it.

The soul is very much dependent on the spirit for its existence.

The soul, the source of emotion, the psuche or psychi, is the life-giver for the flesh or the body. The body (flesh) is the only visible part of the human, while the soul is often expressed. In the natural order of man, we have developed the mindset of looking after the body, which is a must but not at the cost of the other two parts. Generation X, Y and Z are particularly into gratification on demand; giving pleasure to the body and satisfying its needs. We spend billions a year in cosmetic and plastic surgeries, but how much do we really invest in our soul and spirit in time, energy, finance and resources.

Without side-tracking the spirit, I want to spend some time looking at the soul. The soul, the intermediary between the spirit and the body. So essential and can be so volatile. Have you ever seen someone so happy one hour and then at breaking point the next (no it's not just your wife or mother)? The body is only responding to what is going on in the soul. Our primary aim is to maintain the soul to achieve the right equilibrium for our lives. That process is only possible in the soul.

The modern society is dealing with a different level of physical and mental health issues putting a strain on our National Health Services. More and more, diagnosis of mental health illness is affecting people as young as primary school age, which would have been unheard of some years ago. The problem is that the soul is out of alignment and seeking equilibrium.

A few months ago, I conversed with two of my siblings, and we were discussing the power of the mind. I have seen people dressed so well, had started their day well, only to collapse after a few minutes' session with a consultant due to a diagnosis. The strange thing is that, often, the symptoms of that illness will start to show from that point. The secret is the soul.

There is only so much the body can physically do, if the soul (mind) is not involved. I have heard a lot of preachers say that the mind is the most significant battlefield. Most people are caught amid wars and battles even though they appear elegant. The raging storms in the mind, the uncertainty about life and events, the constant demand and needs, can often suppress the ability of the soul to keep going.

The body is subjected to the state and conditioning of the soul. Have you ever seen someone so outwardly beautiful with an appalling attitude? That is not a function of just the flesh; instead, the soul is showing up in our visible realm of the body. Everything you can imagine takes place in the soul; death, life, love, sickness, health, wealth, belief, pleasure, desires, and so on.

The soul is beautifully designed and purposely equipped for what life will throw at us, but the mind cannot function in a void. Everyone must learn the art of mastery over his or her mind.

SOULHARBOUR

One of the most essential things in managing the mind and bringing it in alignment is to set up harbour and ports for the soul.

For those who are familiar with the coast or beach, you will notice the harbours somewhere along the beach where ships and boats can take refuge in stormy weather. This harbour can be so vital for vessels and ships when the waters become contrary. The truth is your soul is not designed to sail through every weather as it will. The mind needs a place to take shelter, and a port to load and unload when it becomes burdened with the vicissitudes of life.

No matter how big a ship, boat, the vessel is, it will need an anchor and a port. Imagine a ship that sets sail with no intention ever to stop; it's heading towards destruction. Occasionally, your mind needs a place to wait, to be still, to recuperate and find strength. If you think about it, when was the last time you sincerely gave your mind some space and a break?

Although the anchor is not the centre of attention on a ship, it gives assurance that the vessel can connect to the sea bed to prevent it from drifting away due to wind or undercurrent. It provides safety for the ship that it will stay in place. One thing I find intriguing is that the strength of the anchor must match the size and weight of the vessel. Many of us can point to instances where we drifted from our core purpose. We may have followed the direction of the wind and current because we had little or no anchor to give the grounding and stability we needed. That could have been an absent parent, an insensitive spouse, a teacher that did not care. Whatever will provide you with the level of anchoring your purpose needs must be strong enough to bear your weight and withstand the wind. Here is the question, what or who is your anchor? Does that anchor have the root and capacity to hold?

Talking about finding the right anchor and having something substantial to hold onto. I remember a few years ago on my mission to become healthier, I went for a trial session at the gym. While waiting for the personal trainer, I couldn't help but notice people that were weight lifting at the far end of the room. As the trainer approached, I remember thinking about how easy the people made it look. My immediate instinct was to ask if I could try that out because I wasn't keen on breaking a sweat on the first day. The trainer asked what my goal was and why I was particularly interested in weight lifting. I wanted to avoid saying "because it looks simple", so I went for the "I just want to try it out" line. He got me to warm up and, needless to say, the rest is history, and I've never attempted lifting another weight at the gym. Looking back in hindsight, if my motivation (end goal) was to work on my cardio and build muscle, then weight lifting may have been the ideal. However, my aim was not to become like Johnny Bravo in my physique with so many biceps, so weight lifting was not what I needed.

That experience was necessary to show that jumping into something I have never trained for or can do could have been suicidal. That is what it's like to anchor on someone or something that cannot take you.

We all start life with a blank canvas (mind), and as we grow and mix with other people, the mind picks up on different weights. The weights are things we go through, our experiences, the things we learn and seek after. But the ability of each person's mind varies from one to another, and what breaks one person may not even affect another. It is, therefore, imperative to choose your anchor carefully.

In the modern world, science has paved the way for in-depth knowledge, especially in medicine. Our evolution as a race is mind-blowing. Our technological advancement, the wealth of knowledge available to us at any given time, the incredible abilities doctors have to remove something from the body or put something in. Processes and systems are more efficient and effective; the list goes on. Despite the advancements, we have not been able to grasp the complexities of the mind fully. We can give someone medication to deal with specific symptoms, but doctors have no power to create or remove a soul. The main reason is that that intricate part does not belong to our tangible realm. Let's explore the field of the soul and what affects it.

SOULFOOD

As a young girl, I remember times when expectation has been badly bruised, mainly when we used to look forward to special occasions. It wasn't just because of the socialising, but the array of foods that would be prepared. The tasting was usually left for the adults, so your expectations increase every time they said it was ready and delicious. The older kids served and, you often notice your younger ones eating very slowly and making you jealous of their privileged position. Another painful experience is when you leave food in the fridge expecting to come home, warm and serve the meal. You often find that the food you'd been thinking about all day is no longer available! This is super common in some families, and that mishap could have cost the culprit an arm and a leg. For most, your food has always been respected and you might not know what I am talking about. For the rest of us who have had such instances where time slows down at the realization that the food is gone, and no matter how much you stick your head in the fridge and shift things around, the recognition of the food being eaten by someone else can be devastating.

Imagine what happens to our souls when expectations are broken and dreams shattered so much it feels almost impossible to get them back.

The soul needs to be nourished with nutrients that will allow and enable it to grow. The realm of the soul is the same realm that the spoken word operates in. Words cannot be seen with the eyes, neither can you catch and lock it away. Just like a plant, you must plant the mind in the place where it can draw and absorb minerals. For us to grow and thrive, the words we speak to ourselves and people speak into and over us provide the minerals the soul is drawing from. Many people are born into toxic environments that strips them of nourishment rather than giving them any. It's even more disturbing when someone grows up and stays in a toxic environment. A toxic environment can be bad relationships, work setting, bad habits, systems and beliefs to mention a few. You must learn to break from the poisonous atmosphere that leaves you empty, unsatisfied, worthless and guilty. It's alarming how many people start life with high expectations and the words of teachers, or a close family member can shatter those ambitions in the twinkling of an eye. Logos can often be used as swords against the soul, and the words you speak to yourself can determine how far you go and how it will end.

Hebrews 4:12: - *for the Word of God is living and powerful and sharper than any two-edged sword, piercing even to the division of soul and spirit, and of joints and marrow, and is a discerner of the thoughts and intents of the heart.*

The spoken word carries so much power and weight that it can transform from bad to good and right to wrong. The ability to make alive and to kill lies in the tongue. Proverbs 18:21

If you think about it, the soul gets its energy from words and such words allow the mind to process so many thoughts and enable the soul to be creative. I often notice that people remember what was said more than gifts and presents and more importantly, the things not mentioned. Some are so gifted they can remember every word of conversation you had with them years before and the way it was said. Even in a relationship, you'll have a man say "but I give you everything". The woman would reply "when was the last time we had a conversation" because the soul is hungry and desperate for some nutrients. We will look at the power of open communication later in the book.

If you have grown up on a bad diet of wrong words, the mind needs nurturing to rid it of the previous. Our mind is continually being fed by what we see and hear. The eyes and ears are very powerful gateways to the soul, and those gates must be under your control as much as possible. Some people can manifest things spoken over them or around them easily because the soul is absorbing and acting on the command of those words. Look at patterns of what happens in specific environments. You may suddenly realise that you were fine before someone spoke about a particular condition, only to find yourself symptomatic of the illness discussed.

"Above all else, guard your heart with all diligence, for out of it flows the issues of life" Proverbs 4:23

The third gateway is our sexual organs (yes). One of the most sacred parts of the body is the organs between the legs, designed for marital pleasure, but also provides the place for significant exchange. What do I mean? We live in a world that promotes sexual freedom. That pleasure, as temporary or lasting as it may be, allows the two to share beyond body fluids, but a complete mixing of identity, purpose and every other thing each person carries.

I remember a time when one of my kids wanted to paint a landscape of the garden, and the most important thing for her was the tree. We had every colour except brown for the tree trunk, and yellow was on its last leg. She was absolutely in love with yellow back then, and she intended to make the sky blue with a big sun in the middle. I encouraged her to mix her purple and some of the yellow to get brown for the tree trunk. Out of excitement, she combined all the yellow with purple and got the brown. The realization that yellow was gone entirely was a shock, and she asked me to remove the bright sunny yellow she needed for the sun from the brown. She soon found out that would not be possible. That happens during sexual intercourse, we create an intense mix of everything we have and own with the other person, and that mix cannot be undone. More importantly, yellow is a primary colour, and you cannot create it by mixing two different colours. The danger of mixing so much is that the person that started life as yellow becomes brown and when brown mixes with another colour like blue, you end up with green.

Some people have lost so much of themselves through the combination and trying to get them back to primary will take so much time and effort. Some may never get it back completely. Every blend leaves a residue. With words, you can hold back and refrain what you say to yourself, or walk away when someone is saying something that does not conform to you. But in the place of sexual intercourse, even when love is not a hundred per cent involved, you are mixing everything; nothing is held back.

I want us to look closely at this principle. Some people are designed as an enigma because they have a primary role in this world. They fit no particular shape or way of life because they have a unique purpose. That different way of life is to propel them to see things and achieve a lot. The second category, are people that complement and enhance something already there. These people will not take the lead in primary roles or necessarily start something new. They make a wave and positive impact on what primaries do because they complement and enhance what is already there. You then have space-fillers. Not in a derogatory way, but we need them just as much as the other category of people. Space-fillers are more inclined to take each day as it comes; they avoid too much change and can often be happy to watch. Have you ever ordered something online and find it delivered in a bigger box or packaging than expected? You will notice that the packaging sometimes contains foams and bubbles to keep the order intact. That is essentially the role of space-fillers; they occupy space to avoid damage through movement. As I have said, space-fillers are more inclined to take each day as it comes, they avoid too much change and can often be happy to watch. Space-fillers are mediocre, and they complain a lot. Now, their complaints can be quite useful as it provides ideas and opportunities, which they will not see but others can make use of them. Space-fillers are mostly at the receiving ends of things. Their purpose is to do their bits every day to keep the job moving the way it should. They are the best market because they need others to deliver and meet their needs.

Back to my mixing example, it would be detrimental to have an enigma in a relationship with a space-filler not just on a physical level, but also on the soul tie level. They will become a burden to each other. The enigma will want to explore, make changes, break barriers and enjoy the experience, whereas the space-filler will instinctively try to confine and protect. Here is the question. Are you still your original self? Have you mixed so much you no longer realize the colour you were created to be, or you wanted to be?

That is why a lot of faith-based teachings solicit for sexual intercourse in the confinement of the marriage, where they have the legitimacy to mix and become one with each other. You will notice that couples that have been in a relationship for a long time start to look and think alike after a while.

I love the way Genesis 2:24 puts it

"Therefore shall a man leave his father and his mother, and shall cleave unto his wife: and they shall be one flesh".

The word cleave is so crucial in the context of sexual intercourse because every sexual experience results in a cleaving; holding onto, being joined together and becoming part of. That powerful mixing unifies the two parties so much so that each takes on the other and retrains it beyond that sexual experience. Some people may notice a sudden change in their thought patterns, their behaviours and taste that may not have been there before. The reason for that feeling of depression, anxiety, could be what has been shared with them during intercourse.

Having examined the three gates to your soul, which one is guarding you most and which one is not as effective? Soul ties through sexual intercourse can be broken when you identified how many you need to unpick through. Being realistic and truthful is not supposed to make you feel guilty, but that is a powerful indication that your life is ready to turn over a new leaf. What did you start life as and what were you supposed to become?

REPRODUCTION

One of the main signs of a healthy soul is that it can reproduce. Any living thing that stops reproducing will eventually die out, and the soul must be encouraged to be productive. The productive strength and ability of the soul lie in creativity. Take a moment with me to look at this verse.

Finally, my brethren, whatsoever things are true, whatsoever things are honest, whatsoever things are just, whatsoever things are pure, whatever things are lovely, whatsoever things are of good report; if there be any virtue, and if there be any praise, think on these things. Philippians 4:8

The Important word for me In that verse Is the "think", encourage your mind to dwell and meditate on things that are true, honest, just, pure, lovely, of good report and praiseworthy, because, over time, the mind will reproduce those things. Every one of us can reproduce our mindset through songs, spoken words, coaching, painting, writing songs or making things. When we listen to music or look at art, all we are doing is gaining access to the mind of the person behind the music or picture.

CHAPTER 3

YOU NEED BOTH PAIRS

Have you ever tried walking with one shoe? It can be very uncomfortable. I can only imagine how Cinderella got home with one shoe that night as she raced against the time. The power in your stilettos is patience and purpose. The purpose must be discovered, and we all recognize it at different stages of our lives. Some discover early in their lives, and they have a clear sense of why they are here, others discover theirs after a significant incident in their life. The key is to learn quickly rather than later as it helps with our decision-making. Walking in purpose brings the satisfaction we may not get from other places. People are stuck in roles they don't like and spend the weekend dreading another Monday until they retire or die. It may be hard to accept, but if you're not around, life will carry on, and families and friends will adjust, but your purpose should not die when we exit this world. Our purpose is usually not just about us, it creates a ripple effect and impact on others and helps them to fulfil their mission.

As crucial as the purpose is, it needs patience for it to mature. Sometimes, our purpose reveals itself in stages, and as we go deeper, we experience layers and uncover more details to our role. It requires time because our purpose forces us to get a deeper understanding of ourselves, our feelings and emotions and the process. You cannot overemphasise the need for time and patience before birthing your purpose.

I had to learn the importance of time and patience during my last pregnancy when the consultant told me the pregnancy was not progressing how they wanted it, and I became ill. To continue with that pregnancy, I had to stay in hospital till I had the baby. Although I became seriously ill, I knew every day I kept the baby inside was a significant benefit to her. When I could no longer carry on, I had to make the difficult decision of giving birth prematurely so that

I could save her life and mine, of course. The delight of holding a new baby was phenomenal, but she didn't look like the others when they were born. This one was tiny, not fully developed and ill. I listened as they discussed her vital statistics, inserted tubes and gave instructions. Our time in ICU and SCBU was difficult; having to come back long after I had been discharged was challenging. I lost weight, and I became depressed and ill all because the baby lost time out of the womb.

When purpose is premature, it needs extra work, so timing is crucial in executing your purpose. The process before manifestation is the most challenging part because we all go through issues that make us ask "why me". Some of us are sitting on experiences that may be the wisdom someone else needs so they need not repeat the process the way we did.

Your process is your story, how you survived, how you made it, and how you conquered. Your process is as vital as your purpose, and you need to develop patience and contentment that while you are going through, you are adding to your knowledge and experience. Drawing on my personal experience, every labour is as unique as the pregnancy. The end result is the same, but the time it takes, and the experience will differ significantly.

FINANCE

We cannot achieve a proper balance if our finance is not adequately dealt with and handled with wisdom. Money is an essential liquid part of life we cannot omit. As women, we need some security around finances and even if you're not there, it's something you can plan and work towards. One income stream is not sufficient even if it brings in more than what you need at the moment. As the saying goes, the trick is not to work harder but smarter.

When we go back to the book of Genesis 2:5 "before any plant of the field was in the earth and before any herb of the field had grown. For the LORD God had not caused it to rain on the earth, and there was no man to till the ground; 6. But a mist went up from the earth and watered the whole face of the ground".

There are a few principles we should consider when developing our financial strategy.

First, choose a day to work on something related to your purpose out of the week. In the above scripture, the Lord held back rain and gave a mist instead of rain because the man had not taken his place in purpose. Many people only experience the mist level of blessing and breakthrough because they are not working on their purpose. The mist level provides comfort and just enough. The rain comes when the place of purpose is occupied.

Second, avoid eating your seed, but learn to sow it back. Cultivate the habit of putting ten per cent of your earnings into something that will yield. For those with tight finance, start with a small percentage and work your way up. Investment can be daunting when we start out, and if you're like me, I need something that speaks plain English so I can grasp it. Attend a workshop, or do your own research and start with a small percentage.

Third, the principle of giving should not be overlooked. I am a firm believer in giving because, when you give, you make room to receive more and it's also part of your process.

Fourth, budget wisely. We all go through different seasons at different times. Your aim in purpose is not to compete with anybody else, so it is vital to learn contentment. We must learn to celebrate the season we're in and be grateful for what you have. Remember that your harvest is still coming.

Last, know that wealth is not only a by-product of hard work alone but following principles that will enhance favour. This is not to undermine hard work, but practical hard work should be based directly on our purpose. Favour brings chances and opportunities which you must identify and grab. Ecclesiastes 9:11

Men, what makes you a husband is not the function of one organ. The woman in your life craves stability and assurance she will be looked after physically, emotionally and financially. If your wife stays at home looking after the children, the sacrifice is not just for now; not having enough disposable income to do the things she may like to. It affects her pension and retirement. As glorious as you may think it is to stay home and look after children, it can be mentally draining and financially frustrating. You have a duty of financial care towards that woman, and you can discuss and agree on what you can do to help out. A lot of women find that stress levels increase during the time of the month when bills must be paid, and the constant checking of the phone may not just be that she's checking WhatsApp status. When her mind is busy calculating where the remaining money will come from and she is logging into internet banking, your well-meaning advances at that time of the night might be met with "what's wrong with you"?

PAIR WITH YOUR PARENT/S

One thing we cannot choose is our parents, and regardless of our relationship with them, they have influence over our destiny. Regardless of what role they may have or have not played, you have a duty of care to them as long as they live. What you do to your parent can often determine how your children will deal with you. The dynamics between parents and children have changed so much; for example, back in the day, parents were consulted before children made significant decisions regardless of how old they are. For instance, in some cultures, marriages are arranged for the children. In some Yoruba cultures and practices, the husband's father will give names to the children of his sons as long as he's alive, but modern culture has changed those practices. I am not necessarily soliciting for that but drawing an example to the shift in our perceptions.

One thing I want to highlight is that our economic position or achievement is not a licence to side-track or demean your parents. Many young people are stagnated due to the way they have treated the channel through which they came into the world. I notice how some young people intentionally ignore their parents. Some are short-tempered and often engage in arguments with their parents. Many are convinced that parents are no longer relevant because we have the use of google. Others have allowed their spouse to come between their relationships with their parents. No matter the offence from your parents, you can still honour them. The power of praying parents is mighty and can open doors and push us ahead.

In John chapter 2, we see the account of the first miracle performed at the marriage feast in Cana of Galilee, where Jesus turns water into wine. I find it interesting that the mother of Jesus went to Him and said they had run out of wine. Even though Jesus essentially told her His time hadn't come,

His mother Mary turned to the servants and told them to follow His instructions. Her action gave Him no choice but to perform the miracle they so much needed and positioned Him for the start of His ministry. Our parents can be so useful in identifying our skills and gifts, so when we are ready for launch, they are best positioned to reinforce our purpose. I want to encourage you to seek the wellbeing of your parents and do things that will make them pray for you.

If you are a parent (grandparent) reading this, it is never too late to build bridges with your children. Generation Y and Z needs parents that can prevail in prayer to effect a positive change in our society. Your role as they get older is that of friendship and advice so you maintain the sacred relationship between both of you. Your task is not to make them a mini version of yourself or force them to do your will, but to encourage them to pursue their goal. Cultivate the habit of praying for them and speaking a positive word over them. Your child/ren need your good wishes.

CHAPTER 4

MAN WITH A MANDATE

I knew the ladies will read this chapter, so as I address this, I am hoping that it will open up the communication channel between you and your lady.

It is incredible that the more we amass, the more polarized many couples subconsciously become. One of the main factors is that we can no longer understand each other as effectively. As I write this, I humbly remember a close friend, who although wasn't much of a talker, was known for his vast wisdom when a matter was discussed with him. I had spent the first few years of our friendship teasing him he left heaven before God could open up his vocals completely. As the years went by, his insight and wisdom were profound, his voice of reasoning was the one many who were intelligent enough would listen to last. I had to take the time to figure out what his secret was. He would allow you to talk and only ever interject one or two important words you'd mention and then listened attentively back to you. Sometimes he would ask a question that would force you to say out loud what you did not intend to say and then create an awkward silence to force you to reflect.

When I summed up the courage to tell him he didn't rush away from heaven and asked him how he does it, he explained that wisdom demands you listen to what is not said as it can often be as important as what was said. A sure sign of maturity is in our communication. When we can break the habit of listening to give a reply; instead to engage the mind, then we improve our communication skills.

Traditionally, meal times were necessary for the family; the time to joke and laugh, talk about the day, help in the kitchen and most importantly listen and understand one another. An African proverb says when the street deals harshly with someone, it's the home that mends them. The house should be our safe haven, a place of freedom and love. That is one reason why the kitchen is the heart of the home. If you're struggling with communication in the relationship, you'd be surprised how even cooking a meal with that person will facilitate the start of a conversation. In most homes, meal times are solo, sometimes in front of the TV or individual rooms, but the roles we play in each other's life remain essential.

If we consider the beginning man, Adam, made in the very image of the Father with very similar characteristics and attributes. In love, God had provided for his health and wellbeing in every possible way. He had a beautiful garden, dominion over every living thing, enjoyable work and the very presence of Yahweh. What Adam had was perfect, but something in Adam was not wholly perfect. He was lonely. There was only so much God could fulfil for this mortal residing on a planet He made explicitly for flesh. God's wisdom to create the woman was to fill the void in Adam's heart. Eve's role in the life of Adam is still pretty much what every woman will long and desire to do for the man that wins her heart. Let's look at the role of Eve in more detail. Remember, Adam did not have to find Eve, God brought her to him out of His love. Eve was handpicked, handmade and hand-delivered by God Himself. Every man that can find that particular woman must understand that only the favour of God makes two people connect in that way. The way their heart can become united, in sync and harmony, can only be through favour. I love the way Proverbs puts it.

"He that finds a wife finds a good thing and obtains favour from God"

Proverbs 18:22

One of the key things to identify with your spouse is what she is in your life. Finding the right person is the deal-breaker. If you indeed found the right one, then realize that you received favour, a privilege.

Adam started life not having to speak until the cool of the day when God visited him. The animals and plants were incomparable to him, no one else to relate with him until God comes later on. Eve was designed to meet the needs of Adam and complement him. One of the critical components of the woman is her ability to talk and relate with Adam differently to the way God speaks with him. This woman was designed to specification; taken from the part closest to his heart, able to get him, understand him and match his thought processes. She could influence and persuade him. She could comprehend him, understand his heartbeat and to support him, not out of chore or duty but out of desire.

In Genesis 3:16, one curse placed on the woman is that the desire of the woman will always be for her husband, and he shall rule over her. That is why I said the innate natural position of the woman is to crave the one she loves and, because of that, she can submit to his rulership. The ultimate way to a woman's heart is in the intimate communication she can have with the man. I am not saying that love at first sight is impossible, but for the woman, the desire grows through communication.

In similar cultures to mine, I often noticed how men are viewed as the ultimate in decision making in the major things around the home. There is a saying I struggled with when I was growing up because I felt it was often used out of context and generally directed at the woman. The adage says "the woman must not cook the stew that the husband does not eat". I thought it was just logic that the woman would not waste her energy cooking something that the husband does not like. I often questioned this notion at the back of my mind. What if she's allergic to what he likes, would she have to cook two meals, for example? But growing up, I soon realized that it wasn't only limited to food but was designed as an all-encompassing rule for the wife. She should not eat, wear and do what the husband does not approve of. The man is the authority in the home, and his wish is a command.

There are countless numbers of women that live their life totally by that rule because, once the heart of the woman truly loves, then her desire aligns with the wish and command of the man.

That alignment does not happen overnight, so you must be patient. The idea is even more challenging when you consider that we are raising girls to value and respect themselves and encouraging them to live life to the fullest. I do not believe that the difference in chromosomes was intended to make one person less relevant. Instead, it facilitates the different roles, where each person can freely express themselves rather than being oppressed by the other. That plays a significant reason in the woman's mind when faced with challenges in her marriage. Often, she cannot walk away because of the children, and second, she loses respect in society because of whatever made her leave home. I pay tribute to the perseverance of women that died because of abuse in their home. Women that never got to see their children become responsible and accomplished adults, women that did not eat the fruits of their hard work. I commend the ones that are alive but broken, damaged, mentally unstable and often side-tracked because of the hardship they faced. Marriage was never designed to frustrate either person. I am certainly not advocating separation or divorce, but when a relationship tears down and undermines the existence of either party, then that is entirely against the will of God.

The desire of the woman, although a curse on her, is a blessing to Adam because, naturally, the woman should have desired the Maker (God) absolutely; God will share this desire with Adam. Your God-given position is one you will be accountable for so the place should not be abused.

Let's take a look at the role of the woman.

Back in Genesis 2:18 and 20, the woman is a helper to the assignment of the man. The primary task of Adam is in Genesis 2:15

"And the LORD God took the man, and put him into the garden of Eden to dress it and to keep it".

All that God had created and placed in the garden was a complete package. The man was not to redesign or reinvent but to dress and keep. The wife (helper) was to assist him in doing that effectively. Before evaluating the assignment of Adam, it is noteworthy that a woman thrives in an environment where the man in her life has a clearly defined purpose. Often, we have women that are too loaded, too blessed, too focused and too intelligent to be on a ship going nowhere. That is why every man needs to have his purpose defined before he marries to help the helper identify where she fits in. Some men may read this and feel that their wives have never been helpful or supportive, but if I turned the table around and asked you what did you need help to achieve? I find it incredible that most couples do the exact opposite of things suggested by their partner and would instead get the idea from someone outside of their team. Could it be possible that you had no clear purpose at the beginning or you did not communicate it across correctly?

Help is an act of assisting someone to do something by offering time, skills, energy and resources. Help implies that you are physically not able to fully achieve something without the assistance of someone else. It is possible to burn out your helper when you leave them to do everything by themselves. Let me put this in perspective. Your Eden comes in the form of your home, your business, your ministry, and so on. Help is an act of favour. When you enlist the support of your wife in her energy, strength, skills and resources to help you achieve your desired outcome from your Eden, that help and favour should not be abused but appreciated and maximized. Your wife must hear what she is doing right, how you feel about her being part of your Eden. When help or favour is abused, it can be taken away. That is one of the primary reasons some couples relate like enemies because the favour (the woman) stopped the innate desire to help and support. Again that process does not happen overnight, it is a gradual experience, where she slowly exits your ship without directly saying she's going. I can almost guarantee that, on the wedding day, most women go into the marriage hoping to have a "happily ever after" because women are keen on the display and how everything appears to the world. She desires to have the best Prince Charming and knight in shining armour and both living the fairy tale life she'd imagined since primary school.

It is worth speaking to your favour to see where you both are in your journey. Try and develop an understanding of your support and help. Your wife may not be able to do everything; she may need training and encouragement in certain areas. You must be willing to help so she can be all that she's designed to be. In the book of 1 Peter 3:7 *"Likewise, you husbands, dwell with them according to knowledge, giving honour unto the wife, as unto the weaker vessel, and as being heirs together of the grace of life; that your prayers be not hindered"*.

Going back to the primary purpose of the man to dress and keep the garden, we need to go back to the original Hebrew word for keep, which is Shamar. In Hebrew, Shamar means to exercise considerable or great care over something. I consider this quite similar to the Name of God in Ezekiel 48:35, where God is referred to as Jehovah Shammah meaning "God is there". That name was a positive indication to His people that the presence of God in the city meant that they were preserved from harm as His presence was a defence.

This very attribute of a caring God, ready to defend and save, can be likened to the role of Adam in his domain of Eden. A man should be prepared to protect and fight for his wife. If you find you are not willing to fight and defend that woman, it's a sure sign that something is displaced. Adam was to be there to care for and protect everything in his domain. A lot of men are busy on the street and may God bless their hustle, but the truth is, how much care have you shown to everything under your control? It is possible to care more for something over another, but not to overlook or side-track something in your care. If you have a woman adequately caring for the home and not working, you must ensure she has your full attention throughout the day, not just the cool of the day experience. Communication is vital to avoid growing apart because the long haul can be demanding.

The second task for Adam was to dress it, and in the simplest terms, he was to embellish Eden so much so that God will admire it when He visits in the evening. This creative God had given Adam creative abilities to be used in the garden to add and make it better. When we dress, we are putting materials on the raw material (flesh). Some can do such amazing tricks, depending on the occasion, that makes people comment positively and admire us. The same applies to the home front. Some things in our garden are raw and in need of dressing.

Talking about adding value, some years ago, a friend asked to borrow my car for a night out with few friends. I had to rush around during the day to ensure the vehicle was available later in the day. I handed over the keys and wished her a pleasant time. To my surprise, she came back later than expected the following day and explained they had a fantastic time. My car had the nasty consequence of an ideal time! They had been drinking and eating in the car, all the rubbish was left, and I got the car with only enough petrol to get me to the filling station. There was the part of me that felt like asking why she did not consider it necessary to fill the petrol back to where it was and clean the inside? Men, if God visited your garden this evening, what would you present back to Him? It is an abuse of God's favour for a woman to come into your domain and deteriorate physically, mentally, emotionally and spiritually. I appreciate that life happens, but everything in the life your wife must not run downhill at the same time if you are embellishing her. Have you been able to develop her confidence more than before? Does she dress better? Does she take time off when you are around, has she been able to pursue her dreams and enhance her career? If your wife is the testimony to all other favours, what would her life say about you? Take stock of the value you are adding to the things in your garden and let her be real with you when you discuss it.

It is interesting that every blessing the Lord released in Genesis 1:28 was directed at both the man and woman even though the woman came after the man had been created. There is a spiritual co-carrier of blessings that God intended for us. There is a look, attribute, character made to fit every person's desire; there is no off-specification to anyone God made. You may not have found the person, but there is someone that needs all of you. That person also carries the same level of grace and blessing you both need to fulfil the purpose.

For the ladies reading this, we all have our ideal prince charming, and, sometimes, he does not come in the package we envisage. If he carries the right grace and blessing and meets the specification, then you're more than halfway there. Looks can change and will change, habits can be learned, and knowledge can be gained if the person is willing to do so. If the substance over the life of a person is wrong, then the relationship becomes a burden on both parties.

CHAPTER 5

BLESSED TO BE A BLESSING

A truly fulfilling life is not just about what we own or how much we have. It's what we do with what we have been given and how many people we can impact positively. When you live life beyond you and your family, you position yourself for greater blessing, increase and satisfaction.

Joshua 15:16-19

And Caleb said he that smites Kirjathsepher and takes it, to him will I give Achsah my daughter to wife. 17 And Othniel, the son of Kenaz, the brother of Caleb, took it and he gave him Achsah, his daughter to wife. 18 And it came to pass, as she came unto him, that she moved him to ask of her father a field: and she lighted off her ass; and Caleb said unto her, What wouldest thou? 19 Who answered, give me a blessing; for thou hast given me a south land; give me also springs of water. And he gave her the upper springs and the nether springs.

The above text encapsulates some of the things mentioned in the previous chapter. Israel had experienced great victory over the enemies as the Lord had promised them. Caleb had played a significant role in moving God's people in faith to possess the Promised Land. Because of his character, Caleb asked for the inheritance on the hilltop saying, as his strength was as a young man, he was still able to climb the mountains and gain ground at the top in Joshua 14:11-15. I loved the attitude of Caleb and the role he played in the book of Joshua. The book of Joshua is similar to the book of Ephesians as it reflects how we can step into our God-given inheritance through faith. There are things you need to apply your authority over and bring them where you want them to be. Caleb was not moved by the size of his mountain or the frailty of his body. He knew that if his mind could see the victory, he would definitely conquer. Some things will not move, change, appear or disappear until you use your authority.

According to his request, Caleb had been given the cities in the mountain, representing fortress, foresight and dominion. The mountain top denotes a place of safety, a place of better view and strength. Caleb played a unique role in the marriage of his daughter, which every father with a daughter needs to note. Many fathers have overlooked the influence they have on their daughters when they start dating. For the daughter, you are the first male in her life, the role-play experience of what she ought to expect from her husband and what she will look for in her man. I remember a conversation I had with my dad when I was younger. He mentioned that he would prefer to be in the same car with his daughters when they were getting married rather than just walking us down the aisle. He replied that it would be the last time to talk over our decision and to share experiences and tips on a successful marriage. Although the tradition dates to when it was considered transferring the woman as her father's property to the groom. For my daddy, it was his opportunity to look at the groom eye to eye to put the fear of God into him. Unfortunately, I did not have the chance to have him carry out that duty.

For Caleb, it was vital for him to see his daughter married to the right type of man. The standard was a man with a can–do-it attitude, who would be prepared to engage in a battle to have the hand of his daughter in marriage. One would wonder why this was a prerequisite for Caleb? Caleb knew that whatever good thing you desire rarely drops off on your lap without you fighting for it. Second, Caleb knew that the task was possible because he had taken over other cities, even in his old age.

Here comes the favour I was talking about; Caleb's promise to the man that conquers was his daughter's hand in marriage. Such is the favour that the right wife carries. She spoke to her husband and persuaded him to ask her father for more than herself because she knew the father's worth. I wonder what came over the husband that he couldn't ask by himself; instead, Caleb turns to the favour (the wife) and asks what she wanted. If Achsah were not there, the husband would have just visited the father-in-law (Caleb) and gone back empty-handed! If a man ever struggles with a prayer request, he knows where to turn to! Imagine saying to a woman "God has asked us to ask Him for anything, and I am not too sure. What do you think we should ask for"? I can bet you she would have a list in no time.

I want to look at the request of Achsah in more detail.

The first thing she said is "give me a blessing". Her requests were not to benefit her, but her husband, who automatically owned her and everything she had. Generally, in those days, the prophetic declaration was reserved to the point of death. The father would call his children around and tell them how their future would be. Jacob did this in Genesis 49. It's worth noting that this blessing was usually reserved for the male children. What Achsah did was to ask for that blessing while Caleb was still agile, sound and audible. She keyed herself into the inheritance of her father so early on that no one would have been able to dispute it with her.

Spiritually, she made the husband benefit from the prophetic declaration of the blessings in Caleb's life. Also, those transferred from his ancestors that only his biological sons should have been entitled to. Ladies and gentlemen, the moment we enter into that marriage covenant and say "I do", we take on so much more than just a name or identity. We become tied to generations of patterns, colours, events, pronouncements, decrees, blessings, curses, and so on. Your children are born into it, your grandchildren will carry it and so on. The most bizarre thing is that we don't get told, because stories are no longer shared, but that doesn't mean it doesn't exist. If we consider the story of Abraham and Sarah, they both suffered from childlessness. Abraham would come to Egypt and lie that his wife was his sister. About 45 years later, Isaac will repeat precisely the same history. It is not because he did not want to be righteous, but because the foundation for deception had already been laid. That deception would run between Jacob and Esau, Abraham's grandchildren, approximately 70 years later. This pattern would continue in the lives of Jacob's sons when they deceived him about the death of Joseph about 120 years later.

If we consider another example from the experience of David in 2 Samuel 12:10. David had committed adultery and killed the husband of the woman to cover his tracks. God passed judgement over David and his family that "the sword will never depart" from his family. Fourteen generations later, Matthew 1 vs 1 describes the genealogy of Jesus, the son of David. In John 19 vs 33-34, the Bible recorded that although Jesus had already died, a soldier took a spear and pierced the side of Jesus. Logically, using a spear would have been to kill Jesus. But the generational decree of over four hundred years raised its head and would not allow Jesus to go without experiencing the effect of the sword. Imagine that Jesus in all His power as God in the flesh experienced such a pronouncement. I could guarantee that something in your generation will show up at some point in your journey.

The second thing she mentioned was that Caleb had given her a Southland. This is attractive as properties were mainly given to male children, whereas, slaves and maids were given to the female children. People that love nature and gardening are most likely to appreciate the south-facing land more than those with little or no interest in it. The reason is primarily that the south-facing area benefits from a vast amount of light, which helps with the growth of plants. The land is not only for the habitation of human beings, but virtually everything we do and process comes from the ground.

For Achsah to possess a land when other brides were given maids and slaves is impressive as she was keyed into economic growth. Ladies, one thing we must strive for without apology is something that can sustain our economic growth, whether property, land, business or investment. One of the most challenging things for the young people to get these days is getting onto the property ladder, and many are stuck in rent cycles, which we need to break from. One of the primary reasons to break from it is that when we rent, we are borrowing someone else's asset. Regardless of how homely it feels, and the number of pictures hanging on the wall, you are borrowing, and the borrower is always at the mercy of the lender. I rent in London, and while working full time within the NHS some years ago, more than half of my income was going on rent. My homeowner counterparts were spending significantly less than I was, so I understand the cycle very well.

For Achsah to provide what the man should have provided was a phenomenon. In the African community, a man has to ensure that the family has shelter, food and clothing. A lot of things have changed in our landscape. However, it can become significant stress for the woman in the home if she's expected to carry the burden even though the man is there. I am not talking about the occasional financial assistance, but year in, year out. One of the most liberating things for women is having a sense of stability. I encourage you also to find something that will support economic growth and allow you to own something, however big or small.

The last thing Achsah asked for was springs of water. Water represents life for every living thing. As tasteless as it may be, it contains essential minerals necessary to sustain a healthy and balanced lifestyle. Everything we do has an element of water attached to it, whether cleaning, drinking, cooking, and so on. A life that has no or very little water will soon die out. One of my favourite stories is in the book of John 4, which tells the story of a woman that met Jesus by the well. I want to highlight the importance of water and derive some principles from there.

In certain parts of Africa, we have a belief that certain spirits roam the earth when scorching in the afternoon. Consequently, pregnant women are usually advised not to walk around during those hours without attaching particular objects to themselves around the tummy area. It may not just be an African. Genesis 18:1 states "Then the LORD appeared to him by the terebinth trees of Mamre, as he was sitting in the tent door in the heat of the day". So this belief may be reflected in other parts of the world.

We believe that both angels and their counterparts walk around the earth at different times of the day. Although we cannot see them except they make themselves visible, they can alter things at will because they are spiritually stronger than human beings. Jesus, at that point, was both man and God. He was utterly man due to the human feeling of tiredness and hunger he experienced on his journey and had to sit by the well. God because his discourse with the woman showed Jesus had the knowledge of her with no one telling Him. He knew what she needed on a spiritual level and transformed her life.

Women fetch water at daybreak because the water is calm, clean and fresh. It means you can start the day early and finish the chores and cooking in good time. This practice was common during the time of Jesus, where women would have gone to the well soon enough to start the day. There was something in her life that made her delay her start to the day. It was that she was considered an adulterer. I want to submit that she was trying to avoid the gossips and the need to defend herself from the whispers of other women. Avoiding everyone meant she delayed the start of her day till midday when she felt no one would be there to talk to or about her. There may be ladies that can identify with this woman, not because you're adulterous, but because there is a visible challenge or issue that people take pleasure in discussing. I want to challenge you to really take the lid off the things that make delay your start. It could be a challenging child, an abusive partner, or an absolute lack. Morning does not last forever, and the longer you delay, the more difficult starting becomes. The need to wait till afternoon meant she probably hadn't bathed, cooked, eaten and must be thirsty. It was this thirst that Jesus ministered to. She was desperate for the living water that would continually spring forth so she would not need to come back to the well.

Back to Achsah, we have a young lady requesting springs of water that will sustain everything she has and guarantee her peace. That, my friend, is what we are seeking in our journey to balance our lives. The spring water is fresh, clean, balanced, overflowing and therapeutic. I love the way David puts it in Psalms 23:2, "*He leads me beside the still waters*". Where the soul is refreshed, peace is found, strength is renewed. It's incredible to know that increasing water intake can help to rid some minor ailments. What is sustaining you and where are you drawing from? The water represents the undiluted Word of God with the power to cleanse, quench every thirst and keep flowing in us to maintain our equilibrium. Caleb gave Achsah the upper and the lower springs. She drew from something more significant than herself, and we must find something that we can align with and receive from. Some people have vast knowledge you can tap into, some can help you find peace with yourself and give you the refuge you need. Your husband may not be all-encompassing, and frankly, he's not supposed to be. For Achsah, she drew from what her father had laboured for, and her husband was the primary beneficiary. You may not have your biological father, but you can come under a spiritual one. Find someone you can be accountable to, someone that can shield, protect and tell you what you need to hear; someone you can be vulnerable to. Vulnerable not in weakness, but someone who can see you as you are.

Ladies, there is blessing you can connect your man to because you are best placed to attract those blessings. If Othniel was a one-word man, he definitely needed Achsah. What otherwise he got in a day, may have taken years if he had to work for them by himself. This is one favour that pulled in other favours. Men, understand that some things are quicker when your favour is well-positioned, cared for and in alignment with you. I respect Othniel for not allowing his ego to take the better part of him.

There are some cultures and beliefs that try to keep a woman below a man. Some men often struggle to adjust to their wives' being higher in some ways, and I understand that. Some believe that a woman will not be submissive if she earns more, or has higher qualifications and so on, but that could not be further from the truth. There is a saying that the empty barrels make the loudest noise. There are women all over the world higher in some respects, and they never let it get to their head. One thing a woman cannot take away is the spiritual positioning you have in the home. Whatever she has and achieves is an added honour to you and your name. If you genuinely love the wife in your life, you must support her to be the best she can be, that when you present her back to God, He should be happy. Your love must not be oppressive or limiting; it should allow her to discover the full glory within her. Before you go all self-righteous, just examine your motives and response when you discuss her aspirations. What are the things you know she does exceptionally well, but no one else knows? She could be a fantastic cook or one of those people that look for the details, she could be overly clean even with ten children in the home. What does she do, that only you benefit from right now? Maybe you are sitting on one of her greatest assets.

Over the years, I have noticed many couples grow apart once their children got older. The conversation dies, and there is a sense of bitterness because the women feel lost, inadequate, or irrelevant. The primary question is why? Many have invested time, energy and every ounce of resources on the building because they are told that the wise woman builds her house. That notion is true, but many have created and have not really had the chance to enjoy that labour. Some have passed under the strain and burden, and another person is now living in what she built. For those blessed to be alive, some are resentful because they look back and they are miles off their purpose. Others feel there is little to point at in terms of achievements. Let me clarify, the home builder is the woman, but what binds it and keeps it intact is the man; the woman is not designed to do both. What she is building should be guided by the man and must be maintained. The wise woman must make her home, but she must also be built up by herself and the people around her.

Let's consider this in more detail. It is common to find that women are "always busy" especially when the family is still young or when they are single. Being trapped in the busy mode can be detrimental for your physical and spiritual wellbeing, and it is not the plan of God for you to burn out. For those who have experienced that feeling of being tired and exhausted, you will know that it makes you less productive and does not necessarily guarantee satisfactory service.

In the book of Luke 10:38-42, we see the story of two sisters, who were followers of Jesus. Martha represents a lot of Christians in the church who are busy doing things in the name of serving. Service is excellent and needed, but your service should match your capacity rather than a constant strain that will make you grumble. Many people are caught in the tradition of doing Church, rather than growing their relationship with God. For God, our relationship with Him is far more critical than our service to Him. Mary knew that Jesus would not be around forever and instead sat at His feet to learn and receive. If you are active in your local church, take time to refresh, recharge and renew yourself often. When we feel stretched in one area, it can have a knock-on effect on other aspects of our lives, so your service must be coupled with wisdom.

The story of Othniel is an interesting one that we can learn from. After he had fought for his wife, he was a judge and a deliverer of God's people.

"When the children of Israel cried out to the LORD, the LORD raised up a deliverer for the children of Israel, who delivered them: Othniel, the son of Kenaz, Caleb's younger brother."

Judges 3:9

The level of accomplishment he had was by no means accidental. Othniel won the primary battle for his wife, received blessings and then was a judge, and because of him, the land had rest for 40 years. Othniel would have been glad he picked his battle well and went after the right woman. Achsah was not mentioned in the Bible after her father gave her to Othniel, and she received the blessings from her father. But the impact she had on him, that made him rise to a deliverer and judge, is a phenomenon. Not every woman reading this will have a limelight season in front of the whole world. But the truth is you are building a legacy in your home and community, and that legacy will outlive you. So I encourage you to take pride in what you are building, work at it persistently and know that you will be rewarded.

CHAPTER 6

FOR THE WOMAN

Every man wants a good woman and, if possible, the best, because people naturally desire good things. One thing both men and women must learn is submission. Ephesians 5 is an exciting chapter where Paul addresses everyone in the home, and the principle is still relevant. From Ephesians 5:22 down, Paul encouraged the following:

The woman to submit to her own husband in everything and the husband to love his wife as Christ loves the Church. Submission is to yield or accept something from a higher authority. We are permitted to express our opinion, but ultimately, the final decision lies with the man. Men, help us to submit, by showing us you are intelligently leading or that you have considered other factors. Submission is not easy and certainly should not be one-sided.

Sometimes, you, as the father and husband, should submit as well.

Ephesian 5:21 "*Submitting yourselves one to another in the fear of God*".

Trust is a significant factor when it comes to submission. If we as women genuinely love our husbands, then we should build trust in their capacity and allow for errors and mistakes. Only when he has confidence in his authority at home can the man lead in other places. Be careful not to break him down and reduce his aplomb to zero. When advising or correcting, we should do it one on one in love and in private. Open rebuke, however well-meaning, can be damaging to any relationship, and the default position should be to talk it over between the two adults. As a woman, we must not be sucked into micromanaging every single thing on the man's agenda or heart. However great you are at managing people, it is not a duty you need to take on in the life of the man. Allow him to take the lead and prayerfully influence his decision.

CHAPTER 7

KEEP THE K.I.D.S

Many parents would agree that raising children in the 21stcentury is a lot harder than a few years ago, but the reality of young people is also changing. There are a greater need and responsibility to be present and involved in their lives than ever before. I want to address some areas we need to focus on, but every child is unique and must be treated as an individual. Our roles are so dynamic in the lives of the children, and we must have the liquidity of mind to adjust to their level and stage. No single person raises a child/ren alone. The role of both parents is necessary for providing balance for the children. This is the ideal and the biblical principles of God. I know that the ideal may differ from your experience, and if so, you are not alone.

Whenever a child comes into the picture of any relationship, the dynamic of that relationship changes and changes, even more, when you have children from previous relationships. It's easy for children to get caught in the drama and breakdown of any relationship, and they should be safeguarded as much as possible. I used the acronyms K.I.D.S to address the areas of focus to ensure the balance we need. If you're a child reading this section, some things will benefit both you and your family.

KNOWLEDGE AND KINDNESS

In the fast-paced environment we live in, a lot is going on in our society we as parents should not brush under the carpet until it gets to our doorstep. I was alarmed by the number of young people that have lost their lives because of knife crime in the city this year alone. What is fuelling the rise is mostly gang-related, but also there are other factors. I came across a young man some time ago as he was running and pleading for money. To cut the story short, he was caught up with drugs, and he needed to pay for a mishap. The society we live in can become so cruel to young people when they feel the pressure of "feeling cool". That feeling comes with a price tag.

Years ago, our parents never bought the right size for anything, it was always oversized and often without a brand name on it. For example, when I started the first year in secondary school, my blazer was to last four years. You could not buy new shoes, it had to be damaged, and you have to explain why. I thought my parents were fascinating until a friend brought in a pack of vests, and when we rolled it out, she could have used it to cover herself. The crux of it is we got away with it with some bullying. After a while, the bullies got used to it when they realized you had no option or your parents would not succumb to peer pressure. For our parents, as long as it's clean, ironed and useable, you were good to go! Like seriously???

The pressure is a lot different, and you, as a parent, have to keep up. The children have cyberbullying, gangs that want to catch them early, and distractions in school, media and other things to sexualize them before they are even ready. You must create an environment where you can talk things over, and address issues at the mole stage. Create time to attend things with them or drop them off. It's ideal listening to the challenges other parents are talking about and don't judge them but use it as a point of discussion with your children. Sometimes, you might not realize how much your children know, and you must familiarize yourselves with some of those things.

It is worth finding something that your children can engage in and develop their knowledge. Years ago, my mentor said if you desire to build any character in your children, aim to expand their understanding. Make them masters in something they enjoy and build kindness, so they don't take things and others for granted. In Proverbs 4:7, it says *"Wisdom is the principal thing, therefore, with all thy getting get understanding"*.

Imagine if every home taught their children the importance of kindness, then school and society will be a better place. Kids, you must learn how to be kind and not pay back a wrong with another wrong. There are things you can do around the home that will not break you or occupy your whole waking hour. In our quest to finding a balance for our mothers, what can you do to help her?

Try loading the washing machine and pressing the start button or taking the rubbish out. Some of you may have a father who wants everything squeaky clean when he gets home. Try and clean up half an hour before he gets in, so your mother doesn't have to defend the house being messy.

INDEPENDENT AND IMPARTED

Do you remember growing up and wishing you were older than you were? One of the baits is the feeling of freedom and being independent, especially if you grew up in homes with strict rules. For the modern generation, the desire for independence and freedom is ever more pressing. It's so appealing at first, and then they realize the price far outweighs the privilege. One of the biggest challenges for some women is allowing the children to grow beyond the cute baby stage and giving them the room to discover who they are. As caretakers, our primary aim is to love, guide and provide the resources they need to be healthy and fulfilling.

One way to encourage independence is to allow them to participate in things that match their strength, age and ability. At times, we may feel it's easier to do some tasks by ourselves, but learn to step back.

By allowing them to participate in chores around the house, make them clear up, and helping to carry shopping is part of the training. I used to cringe when I asked the kids to clear up or clean the dishes, and one of them would reply "I didn't put it there' or "it's not my turn". I was more upset when I realized the whole argument was over one plate and a teaspoon! I would wash it just to make them stop arguing over something so small. To my surprise, they found something to contend about five minutes later! After ending up in the hospital, tired and exhausted, I played along. When they refuse to wash a few plates and cutleries, I add all the clean dishes and tell them to sort it out. I had to do only it twice. Sometimes you find a small handful of food in a topper ware intentionally left there. This is just to create the illusion there is something in there or avoid washing the topper ware. I devised my own plan to get them out of the habit.

When you allow them to be independent, we are using the opportunity to teach them life skills. Some years ago, I used to prepare a different breakfast for everyone. Now I let them sort it out, and that's the only time we eat different foods. The rule is they must only take out what they can finish, and everyone must clear up after themselves.

Independence must have boundaries, and those boundaries must be stated clearly and discussed. Children must realize that we allow freedom per their maturity and it's not just a given.

DEVELOP

As incredible as we are, we all have areas we need to work on and develop, and personal development should be continuous. By working with our little treasure, we can address weakness one by one and invest in proper training. Work with your children to develop achievable milestones over some time and reward achievements. When my kids were a lot younger, I decided to get them into reading. Everywhere we went, I always tried to carry a couple of books, and I used to read on the train and buses and made it as fun as possible. That was my little way of keeping them quiet when in public but also to help them develop their imagination. These days, we all play games around the books we've read and act out characters and sometimes we have other people join in on public transport. I had an occasion when I had to do the school run with 8 children on the tube and train, and that was the trick I used. We played games, and I intentionally asked them difficult maths questions with a treat for the first person to get it right. I was surprised to see adults trying to help the children get the answer. You may have more exotic methods, especially for other key subjects which you can try out. It adds to the memories and encourages continuous learning, so use every opportunity to develop their social skills and knowledge.

SOCIETY

Many of us grew up on the saying it takes a village to raise a child, and it was so right. If you are a young person reading this, you can count yourself very lucky. We grew up answerable to virtually every adult in the town. You had to behave yourself because other adults could tell you off, discipline you and then tell your parents. I still believe that it takes a village to raise a child.

The modern world is very different, with little interaction between neighbours until something happens. Every human being is limited in one way or the other and raising children cannot be done exclusively within your four walls. That will break you. You must develop your village, your community of people who you trust, people with a genuine interest in the wellbeing of your child to work with. Growing up, whenever my mother disciplined us, her siblings knew about it, and they all sided with her and sang from the same hymn book. They all echoed their principles whether our parents were there or not and that was powerful. There was a constant reminder that someone could catch you doing something and report you. Choose your village wisely—people with similar principles to yours.

I was quite shocked many years ago when a mother abused a teacher because her son was sent out for disrupting the class. Teachers are not angels, and they can sometimes get things wrong. But surely, abusing the teacher in front of her child, other children and parents is inappropriate. When children feel they need not answer to anyone except their parent that is a telltale sign that something is wrong. Our village and community help to build the children for the future and the real world, when mummy and daddy will not be in the boardroom. Children must be accountable to other people outside the immediate family, who want the best for them.

CHAPTER 8

IT'S TIME TO H.E.A.L.

One desire of God is that we come into everything He has created for each of us. 3 John 1:2 is a promise of a loving father that wants our prosperity and good health. In this last chapter, I want to focus on areas that can improve our health and wellbeing using the acronym H.E.A.L.

HEALTH AND HAPPINESS

One thing we cannot put a price on is our health and happiness, and the two should not be taken for granted in our journey. What we feed the body can affect the way we feel and look. You must pay attention to your health and wellbeing and start to make little changes where you can to keep you going. Our foods are produced in ways that maximize profits and often strips the goodness out of the foods we eat.

I want to challenge you to have at least one meal a day you cook from scratch. Fruits, vegetables and herbs are natural medicines our bodies need to fuel our internal system. By introducing these raw ingredients into our diet, we can help our body to function better. If you have a habit of living on caffeine or energy drink, try introducing water in small quantities throughout the day.

Just as our body needs food, our soul also must be fed. Start with things that make you happy. Do you notice what happens when children get Christmas presents? The happiness is often short-lived after the wrapping paper comes off, whether it cost one pound or a hundred pounds. That's because the mind holds onto pain and quickly forget good things. One way to retrain the mind is through the constant reminder of the things that make you happy and the things you are grateful for. We remember pain because we talk about it often to ourselves and to others. Shift your emphasis on the positives, and it may surprise you there are more things to be grateful for than you expected. Try talking happily to yourself at least a few times a day.

EXPLORE

A limited perception hinders foresight. When you explore things around you, it increases your scope and knowledge. Back to my beach scene, many people walk along the seashore, some sit and sunbathe, and some build sandcastles. All have something in common, and that's the sand. The view at that level is relatively limited, and the experience similar. Do you realize those that dare to venture into the sea will have a different experience to the first group? Many have just scratched the surface of their purpose, and have stayed on the sand level too long. I want to challenge you to step into the sea. It could be changing your career, starting a new hobby, gaining your qualification, learning how to drive or just going out to meet new people. You need to step into the sea.

ATTENTION AND ATTITUDE

In the army or police training, there is sometimes the call for attention, where body and focus are at alert. I am making that call to you because you need to focus and be at alert for the greatest battle of your life; the struggle for your purpose. What are you focused on at the moment? Seeing is a function of the eyes, but the focus is of the mind. Your mind must realign to what you are designed to do, not what you are being forced to do. As you realign your perception, your attitude must be disciplined. Your approach is the determining factor in how you sustain the height you attain.

One of the best attitudes we need as we pursue our purpose is humility. In its purest form, we can control our power. As you go further and higher, check the motives behind your actions. It can be something so simple as wearing the costly outfit to oppress someone or talking so it makes another person feel inferior to ourselves. How much can God trust you with before it gets to your head?

LET IT GO

In your pursuit of purpose, you need to identify the unnecessary loads you are carrying with you and how essential they are for your journey. Remember, the soul is not designed to take on everything, and it can collapse under pressure. God delights in our prosperity and advancement, but you can limit yourself when you allow unresolved issues to keep you grounded in the past. The past can have such a negative effect on your development, and you need to learn to reduce the load by admitting what the hurt was. The next thing is to understand the need for forgiveness is not for the other person but for ourselves. Often, we wait for someone to admit something and ask for mercy, but that is a sign of immaturity. Learn to accept that pain and hurt are part of life. The effect is more significant when the pain comes from someone close. You must allow your soul to get rid of it before it takes a root of bitterness. Hebrews 12:14 comes to mind "*follow peace with all men*" because it acts as a shield for your soul. Not everyone is going to reciprocate peace, and this is also normal, but your soul should get to a level where it will not react to certain things. I am working through this, and, at times, it is so difficult because people can be malicious intentionally as everyone seeks their pound of flesh.

Bitterness shows you have attached far too much importance to someone and given them too much power over your soul space. The dominion in your soul should be decided by whatever is sustaining your spirit. Bitterness can lead to health issues and other negative impacts in other areas of our lives. Whatever happens, do not allow pain to change your persona. A Yoruba saying is that "if you close your eyes for the wicked to pass when a good person passes, you will not know". Many people are stuck in a particular season of their lives because bitterness has locked the door to their next season. Many have failed the test of time because they did not conquer the rage of resentment. Unforgiveness has shut the door of opportunities, and, only had they made a move towards reconciliation, things might have turned out differently. There is probably someone else hurting because of you. What you said or didn't tell, the way you looked at them or the fact that you did not respond to their call in time of need. You may not have done it intentionally, but every one of us will have an offence hanging over our head. I want to encourage you, LET IT GO! Forgetting a wrong takes time, but forgiveness does not have to.

LASTLY

Like my mentor advised, there is no manual for everything we experience in marriage, our relationships, career or anything else life may throw at us. We all have our stilettos that only you know how it fits and feels, but the more you master it, the more your feet adjust to it. But everything you need to live and fulfil is right in you and accessible to you if only you are willing to reach out and work for it.

I want to pay something forward to you and hold the door of opportunity open for you just like I experience it. Change can be daunting, and leaving your comfort zone and stepping in the sea, or becoming creative with the need to apologize can seem overwhelming. One of my significant changes was pursuing a long-term goal and writing this book, which I had procrastinated for years. I come to you like the Prince with the lost stiletto to say you can take off the borrowed pair and wear the shoe life intends for you. Your stilettos may hurt to start off with, your flesh will resist anything that takes you from your known and comfort zone towards your perfect position.

One can imagine how people in that town would have reacted to Cinderella when she stepped into her shoes. Her position changed from the lady with rags, the home cleaner, to a princess.

Expect attacks and resistance from people around you that do not believe in your dreams. Avoid those that feel you are not deserving of something better and higher than where you have been. Avoid the voice of your flesh that makes you shut down your ambition and throw in the towel before you have even started. It's time to step in and step up.

EPILOGUE

I have struggled to walk, although not entirely, but to be able to move my physical body from one point to another as I like.

I have struggled to breathe, not an act of pride or right but to maximize every ounce of borrowed time I have.

I owe it to my soul to be free, to be alive in the real sense of living the abundant life in love and all that God has bestowed on me.

My horizon becomes that little bit clearer and the sight of hope, however dim, makes me take that extra step to be myself.

Printed in Great Britain
by Amazon